WHAT!!!

CONSTIPATION

Hale Jones1

Healthy tips on how to be free from constipation

Hale Jones2

Copyright

Hale Jones3

Table of Contents

Hale Jones4

Chapter Four: How is constipation treated under management and treatment?

Chapter Five: What Can I Do To Prevent Constipation?
- Did you know that??

About the Author

Acknowledgement

Special thanks goes to the Almighty who has always been the origin of ideas and wisdom.

To my Parents and siblings, who have always been my source of Encouragement and strength, I will never let you down.

To my Readers, who never give up on trying more ways to achieve a healthy lifestyle, this guide won't be a disappointment, but an informative guide.

Hale Jones6

Introduction

People's ideas of what constitutes "normal" bowel habits can vary greatly.Constipation is therefore one of the most challenging gut symptoms to define.Researchers, patients, and medical professionals all have different perspectives on this condition.

The majority of us occasionally experience constipation.We may experience some irregularity in our bowel movements due to illness, inactivity, travel, medications, and other factors.

This is exemplified by:

sporadic or hard stools that frequently come with abdominal discomfort or even pain, straining, and the sensation of an incomplete evacuation. These symptoms typically last only a short time and do not significantly alter daily life.For some, the first sign of a bowel disease such as diverticulitis or Crohn's disease may be an abrupt onset of constipation. Other examples of

Hale Jones7

obstruction include tumors, adhesions, and inflammation.
Constipation's sudden and persistent onset can be a major concern.If the symptoms include extreme pain, fever, bleeding, or vomiting, you should tell your doctor.

Hale Jones9

CHAPTER ONE

What's constipation?

Constipation is having fewer than three bowel movements per week.
However, each person's frequency of "going" varies greatly.
While some people experience bowel movements on a daily basis, others only once or twice per week.

Constipation is one of the signs of dysfunction in your outlet.
Remember to discuss your bowel movements, questions, and concerns with your doctor openly and honestly. We ought to all poop at some point. Constipation can be a sign of a more serious condition, a temporary issue, or a problem for a long time.

Whatever your pattern of bowel movements is, it is individual to you and normal, as long as you don't go too far from it.
Hale Jones10

One thing is certain, no matter how your bowel movements are going: Stool or poop passes more difficultly the longer you wait before "going." Other important characteristics that typically define constipation are:

- You have hard, dry stools.
- Your bowel movements are painful, and it's hard to pass your stools.
- You feel like you haven't completely emptied your bowels.

Is constipation common?
If you suffer from constipation, you are not alone. In the United States, constipation is one of the most common gastrointestinal complaints. Constipation brings at least 2.5 million people to the doctor each year.
Constipation can occur on occasion in people of any age.

Consistent constipation, also known as "chronic constipation," is also more likely to occur in certain situations and with certain people.
Hale Jones11

These are some:
Greater age
Compared to younger people, older people tend
to be less active, have a slower metabolism, and
have weaker muscle contractions along their
digestive tract.

**Being a woman, particularly during
pregnancy and postpartum.**
Constipation is more common in women who
experience hormonal changes. Squeezing the
intestines while the baby is still inside the womb
slows down stool flow.

Not getting enough foods high in fiber.
Foods high in fiber speed up the digestive
process.

Hale Jones13

CHAPTER TWO

What causes constipation?

Your colon absorbs too much water from waste (stool or poop), which dries out the stool and makes it hard to push out of the body and causes constipation.

To recap, nutrients are typically absorbed as food moves through the digestive tract. Waste, or food that has only been partially digested, moves from the small intestine to the large intestine, also known as the colon.

The solid matter known as stool is produced when the waste is soaked up by the colon with water.

Food may move through your digestive tract too slowly if you have constipation. The colon has an excessive amount of time to absorb the waste's water as a result of this. Pushing the stool out becomes difficult as it becomes dry and hard.

Food waste pathway through the rectum, anus, and colon.

Hale Jones14

Is it possible for constipation to result in internal damage or other health issues?
If you don't have soft, regular bowel movements, you could end up with some problems. Some problems include:

- Hemorrhoids, or swollen, inflamed veins in your rectum, are a condition.
- Anal fissures are tears in the lining of your anus caused by hardened stool trying to pass through.
- Diverticulitis is an infection that occurs in pouches that occasionally form off the colon wall as a result of infected stool that has become trapped.
- Fecal impaction is the accumulation of too much feces in the rectum and anus.

Struggling to move your bowels can cause damage to your pelvic floor muscles. Your bladder is controlled by these muscles.

- Stress urinary incontinence is a condition in which the bladder leaks urine after too much straining for too long.

Hale Jones15

**Is it possible for me to become ill if I don't
have regular bowel movements?**
Don't worry; this rarely happens.
Constipation causes your colon to retain stool
for longer, which can make you feel uneasy.
However, the colon is an expandable container
for waste. If waste gets into a wound that is
already there in the rectum or colon, there might
be a small chance of getting a bacterial infection.

Hale Jones16

Hale Jones17

CHAPTER THREE

Constipation symptoms and causes.

What causes them?

Constipation can be brought on by a variety of factors, including lifestyle choices, medications, medical conditions, and pregnancy.

Constipation can occur for a variety of reasons, including:

- Consuming foods that lack fiber.
- Insufficient water intake (dehydration).
- Not enough physical activity.
- Alterations to your usual routine, like eating or traveling at different times or going to bed at different times.
- Consuming a lot of cheese or milk.
- Stress.
- Being unable to resist the urge to urinate.

What symptoms does constipation present?

The following are signs of constipation:

Hale Jones18

- You void less than three times per week.
- Your stools are dry, lumpy, or hard.
- It is difficult or painful to pass your stools.
- You feel cramps or a stomachache.
- You feel nauseated and bloated.
- After a bowel movement, you feel as though you haven't completely emptied your bowels.

CHAPTER FOUR

How is constipation treated under management and treatment?

Self-care: You can usually treat mild to moderate constipation at home.The first step in self-care is to make changes to your diet and lifestyle.

The following are some suggestions to ease your constipation:

- Each day, consume two to four additional glasses of water.
- Avoid beverages with caffeine and alcohol, which can dehydrate you.
- Include whole grains, fruits, vegetables, and other high-fiber foods in your diet.
- Reduce your intake of high-fat foods like cheese, eggs, and meat.
- Consume bran cereal and/or prunes.
- Keep a food diary and focus on the foods that cause you to bloat.
- Move around and exercise.

Hale Jones20

- Examine your toilet seat position: It may be easier to urinate if you squat, lean back, or raise your feet.

Hale Jones21

CHAPTER FIVE

What Can I Do To Prevent Constipation?

You can prevent constipation from becoming a long-term issue by continuing to treat it at home using the same methods:

- Consume a well-balanced diet high in fiber.

 Whole-grain breads and cereals, legumes, fruits, and vegetables are all excellent sources of fiber. The colon uses fiber and water to pass stool. Apples, for example, have skins that contain the majority of their fiber.

The most fiber is found in fruits that have seeds that you can eat, like strawberries.

Bran is an excellent fiber source. Consume bran cereal or add bran cereal to yogurt and other dishes. Between 18 and 30 grams of fiber should be consumed daily by people who suffer from constipation.

- Every day, consume eight 8-ounce glasses of water.

Hale Jones22

Did you know that??

- Constipation can be caused by milk in some people). Coffee and soft drinks, both of which contain caffeine, can dehydrate you. It's possible that you'll need to stop drinking these things until your bowel movements get back to normal.

- When you feel the need, move your bowels. Do not delay.

Hale Jones23

About the Author

Hale Jones is a Nutritionist and someone who is Keen on personal development.

Hale Jones24

www.ingramcontent.com/pod-product-compliance
Lightning Source LLC
Chambersburg PA
CBHW051729250726
48653CB00008B/3274